Ebola (Ebola Virus Disease)

The Facts and Fiction about a Rare and Deadly Disease

Copyright © 2014, Owen Williams

All rights Reserved. No part of this publication or the information in it may be quoted from or reproduced in any form by means such as printing, scanning, photocopying or otherwise without prior written permission of the copyright holder.

Disclaimer and Terms of Use:

Effort has been made to ensure that the information in this book is accurate and complete, however, the author and the publisher do not warrant the accuracy of the information, text and graphics contained within the book due to the rapidly changing nature of science, research, known and unknown facts and internet. The Author and the publisher do not hold any responsibility for errors, omissions or contrary interpretation of the subject matter herein. This book is presented solely for motivational and informational purposes only.

Table of Contents

Introduction	4
Ebola: What is it?	5
The First Case of Ebola	6
Bats as Carriers for Ebola	8
Signs and Symptoms of Ebola	10
How is Ebola Diagnosed?	12
How is Ebola Transmitted?	14
Risk of Exposure to Ebola	16
Treatment for Ebola	17
Prevention of Ebola	19
Past and Present Outbreaks	21
Ebola Q&A	25
Conclusion	27
Photo Credits	28

Introduction

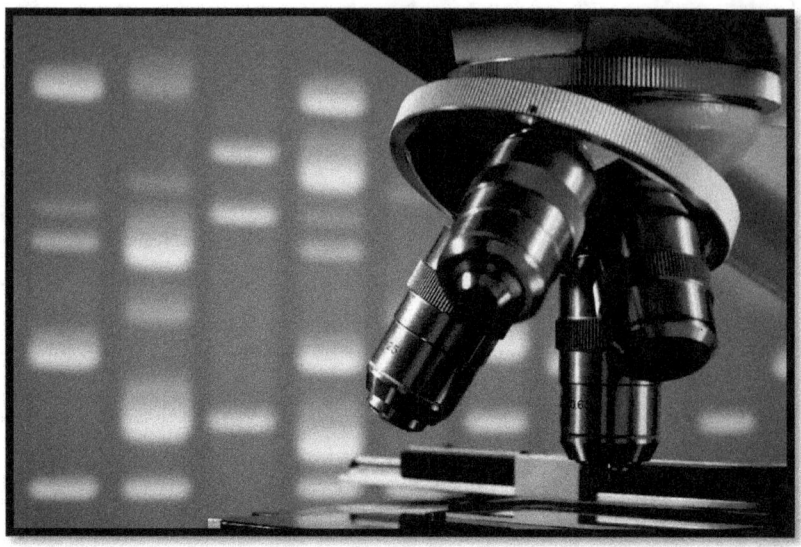

      Ebola, or Ebola Virus Disease, is an incredibly dangerous and deadly disease. What many people do not realize, however, is that this disease is also very rare and your chances of contracting the disease are slim unless you come into direct contact with the blood or bodily fluids of someone showing symptoms of the disease. In order to protect yourself and your family, it is recommended that you learn as much as you can about this disease and that you avoid spreading false information yourself. That is where this book comes in. In this book you will learn the basics about Ebola including what it is, how it is diagnosed, and what the treatment options are. By the time you finish this book you will have a basic understanding of this deadly disease so you can help to stop the spread of misinformation and keep your family safe from the disease.

Ebola: What is it?

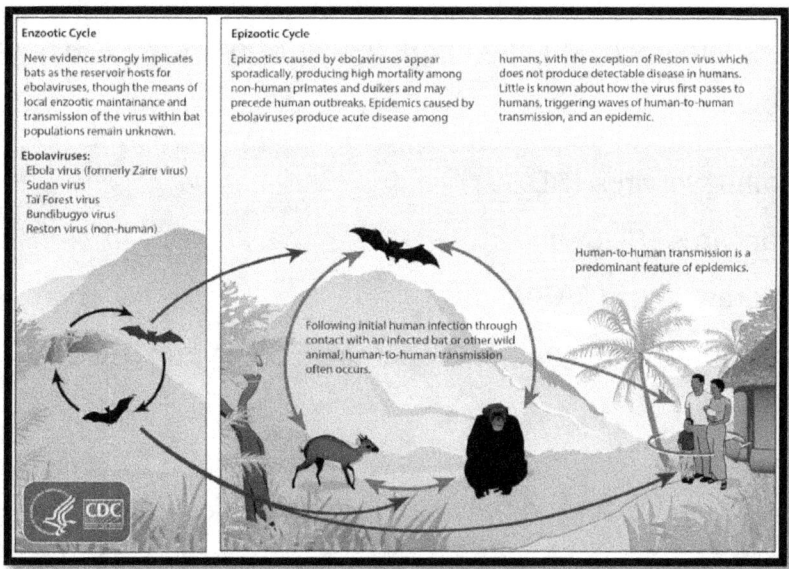

Though the official name is Ebola Virus Disease, the illness caused by the Ebola virus is typically referred to simple as "Ebola." This disease first appeared in Africa in 1976 with two outbreaks occurring in different parts of the continent simultaneously. Ebola is a rare but extremely deadly disease that is caused by the Ebola virus and it is passed through direct contact with bodily fluids (including blood) of an infected person – more specifically, of someone who is already showing symptoms.

Before you can understand how Ebola affects humans, it may be worth learning where the disease comes from and how humans first contracted it.

The First Case of Ebola

The type of Ebola that infects humans comes from four out of five strains of Ebola virus – that is, viruses belonging to the genus *Ebolavirus*. <u>The names of these viruses are as follows</u>:

- Bundibugyo virus (BDBV)
- Sudan virus (SUDV)
- Tai Forest virus (TAFV)
- Ebola virus, formerly known as Zaire Ebola virus (EBOV)

Though Ebola can be spread between humans by contact with the bodily fluids of an infected person, it is unclear how the disease first came to infect humans. The first case of Ebola to affect humans is thought to have been transmitted through contact with an infected wild animal – possibly a fruit bat. Though bats are one of the animals most likely to carry Ebola virus, other possibilities include several species of monkey including gorillas, duikers, baboons, and chimpanzees.

Animals can become infected with Ebola virus when they eat fruit that has been partially eaten by a fruit bat carrying the virus. There is some evidence to suggest that both domesticated pigs and dogs can be infected with Ebola virus. Because dogs typically do not develop any symptoms of the disease it is unknown what role they play in spreading the disease to humans. Pigs are at least known to be able to transmit the disease to primates.

As it has been mentioned, the origins of the virus are unknown but fruit bats are the most likely candidate for being the "natural reservoir" for the Ebola virus. The term "natural reservoir" is given to the long-term host of an infectious disease or pathogen – in most cases, the host does not contract the disease, it is merely a carrier. Identifying and studying the natural reservoir of any given disease makes it possible to study the life cycle of the disease and to develop prevention and control methods. Because it has not been officially confirmed that bats are the natural reservoir for Ebola, prevention and control methods are still being developed and studied.

Bats as Carriers for Ebola

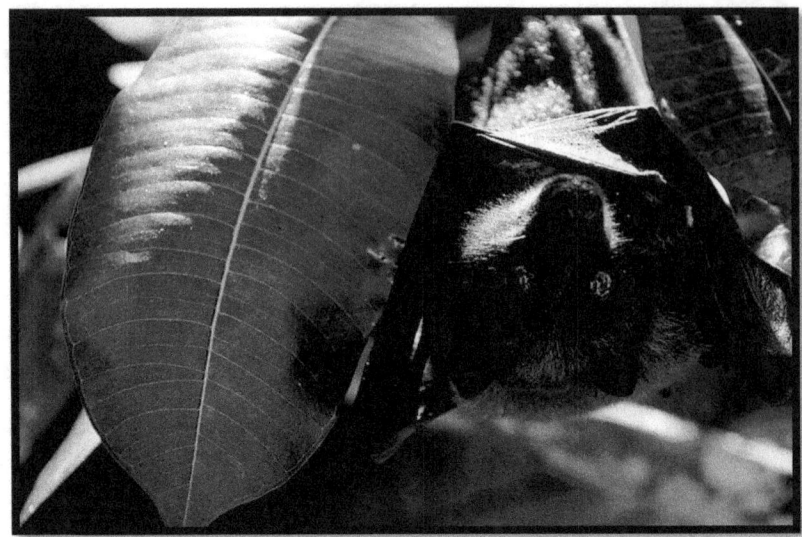

There are three different types of fruit bat that have been identified as being able to carry the disease without contracting it. These species include:

- Hypsignathus monstrosus
- Epomops franqueti
- Myonycteris torquata

Though certain plants, birds, and arthropods have been considered as possible natural reservoirs for the virus, as of 2013 it is still unknown whether other species of animal have been involved in the spread of the disease. The fact that bats were found roosting in the cotton factory where the first case of Ebola originated supports the theory that bats are the natural reservoir for the disease.

In order to test the likelihood of bats being the natural reservoir, scientists inoculated 24 different plants and 19 animal species with the virus. The only animal or plant to become infected was the bat and, because it showed no clinical signs of the virus, this further supports the theory that they are the natural reservoir for Ebola virus disease. Upon further inspection, antibodies for both Reston and Zaire viruses were discovered in fruit bats – this adds to the scientific evidence in support of the theory. Other tests have been conducted on various species of rodents but there is little evidence to suggest that they are the natural reservoir for the disease.

Signs and Symptoms of Ebola

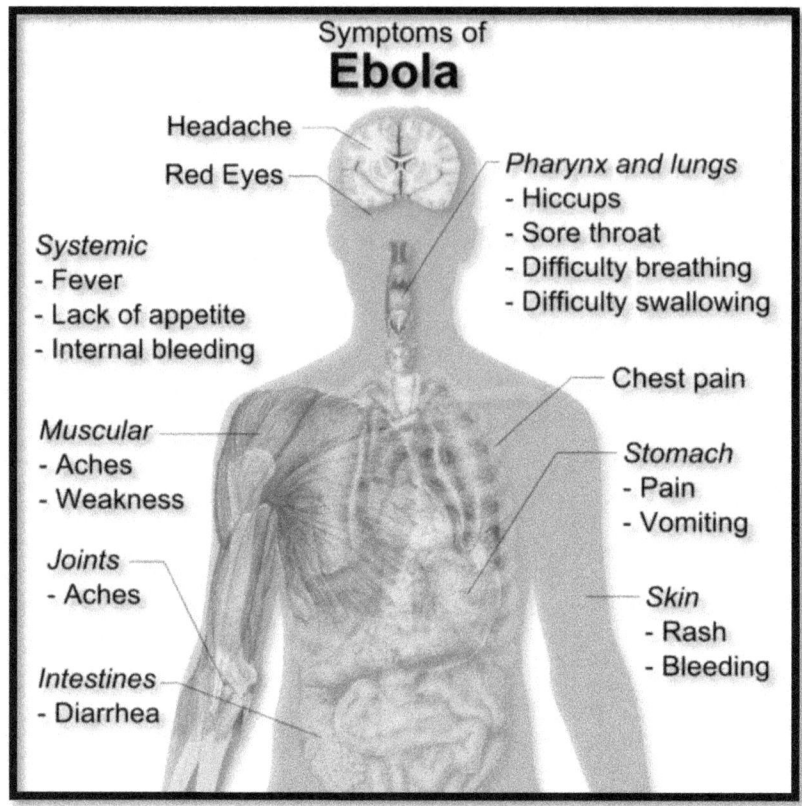

Perhaps one of the trickiest things about the Ebola virus is that there is an incubation period of the disease lasting between 2 and 21 days. This means that an individual could become infected but might not start showing outward symptoms for as long as 3 weeks after contracting the disease. It is important to note that humans cannot transmit the disease – they are not considered infectious – until they start to display outward symptoms.

Some of the symptoms associated with Ebola include:

- Fever
- Fatigue

- Muscle Pain
- Headache
- Sore Throat
- Vomiting
- Diarrhea
- Rash
- Impaired Kidney/Liver function
- Internal or External Bleeding
- Low White Blood Cell Count
- Elevated Liver Enzymes

Ebola has the potential to manifest in different ways in different people. For the most part, however, the first symptoms an infected person develops include fatigue, fever, headache, muscle pain and sore throat. As the disease progresses, the individual may experience diarrhea, vomiting, and rash – some also begin to display outward signs of liver and kidney impairment. In some cases, individuals may even experience excessive bleeding (either internal or external) in the form of bleeding gums, blood in the stool, or other forms of bleeding.

How is Ebola Diagnosed?

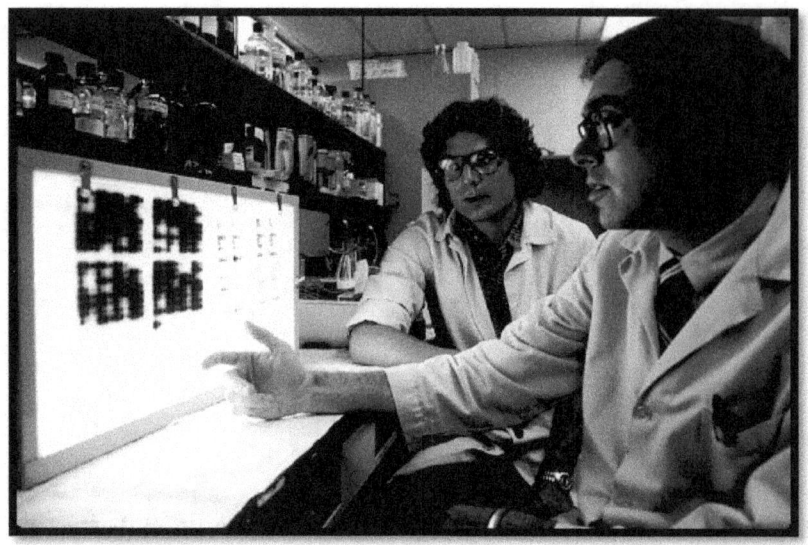

Because the symptoms of Ebola are very similar to the symptoms of other diseases including meningitis, malaria, and typhoid fever, it can sometimes be difficult to diagnose. Ebola is a very rare disease so, unless you have been exposed to someone who is symptomatic and have had contact with their bodily fluids, your doctor is unlikely to suspect Ebola over the three diseases previously mentioned. Diagnosis for Ebola cannot be made by observation of symptoms alone – <u>there are certain laboratory tests that must be taken, including</u>:

- Antigen-capture detection test
- Antibody-capture enzyme-linked immunosorbent assay (ELISA)
- Serum neutralization test
- Electron microscopy
- Reverse transcriptase polymerase chain reaction assay (RT-PCR)
- Virus isolation using cell culture

Diagnosis within the first few days of developing symptoms is very difficult and only certain tests will be effective until the disease has progressed a bit more. <u>The tests which can be administered during the first few days of symptom development include</u>:

- Antigen-capture detection test
- Antibody-capture enzyme-linked immunosorbent assay (ELISA)
- Reverse transcriptase polymerase chain reaction assay (RT-PCR)
- Virus isolation using cell culture

Once the symptoms develop further, the patient can be tested for IgM and IgG antibodies to confirm a diagnosis. If the patient dies as a result of the disease, postmortem tests including immunohistochemistry tests, PCR, and virus isolation can be used to confirm the diagnosis.

Because samples from patients infected with Ebola are a high biohazard risk, the samples may need to be transferred to and studied in an area where biological containment measures are being put into place. If the patient has started to show symptoms and if it has been confirmed that the patient came into contact with the bodily fluids of an Ebola-infected person, that patient should be immediately quarantined and the proper tests taken to confirm diagnosis.

How is Ebola Transmitted?

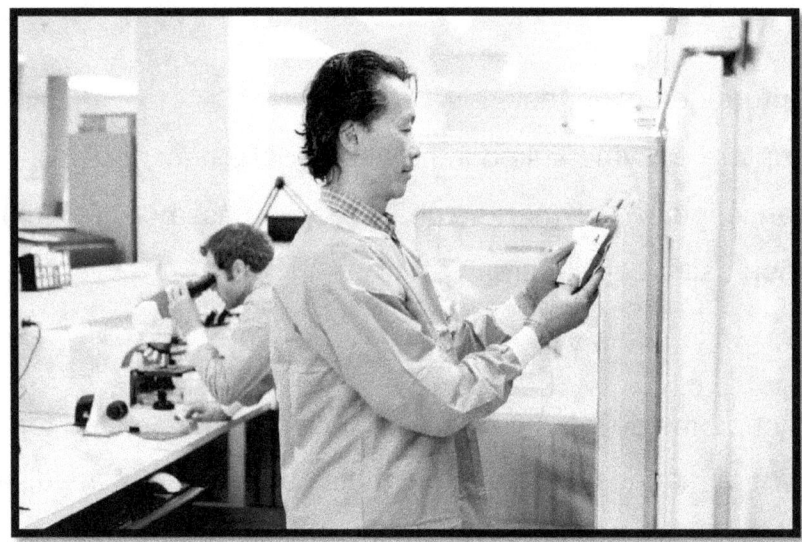

The transmission of Ebola is not yet fully understood because the natural reservoir for the virus has yet to be confirmed. Though the origins of the first case of outbreak in humans is unknown, scientists have confirmed the ways in which one human can transmit the disease to another. There are several ways in which the virus can be spread between humans:

- Direct contact with blood or bodily fluids of a person showing symptoms for Ebola (saliva, urine, feces, sweat, vomit, semen, and breast milk)
- Direct contact with objects that have been contaminated by the Ebola virus (ex: syringes and needles)
- Contact with infected primates or fruit bats

It is important to understand that Ebola is not transmitted by air, water, or food. In Africa, however, there is some evidence to suggest that the virus can be transmitted through the handling of bushmeat. There are only a few species of animals which have been identified as being capable of becoming infected – mosquitoes and other insects cannot transmit the virus to humans.

During an Ebola outbreak, the virus can spread quickly if proper control methods are not taken. Exposure is particularly likely for hospital staff who come into contact with an infected patient while not wearing the appropriate protective equipment (this includes gloves, gowns, masks, and eye protection). Family and friends of an infected person are also at risk if they come into contact with the patient's bodily fluids. Because the disease can be spread so easily in a hospital environment, hospitals often use dedicated (ideally disposable) equipment to treat Ebola patients.

*Note: Once a person recovers from Ebola, they are no longer capable of transmitting the disease to others. It has been found, however, that the Ebola virus can be spread through the semen of a recovered person for up to 3 months.

Risk of Exposure to Ebola

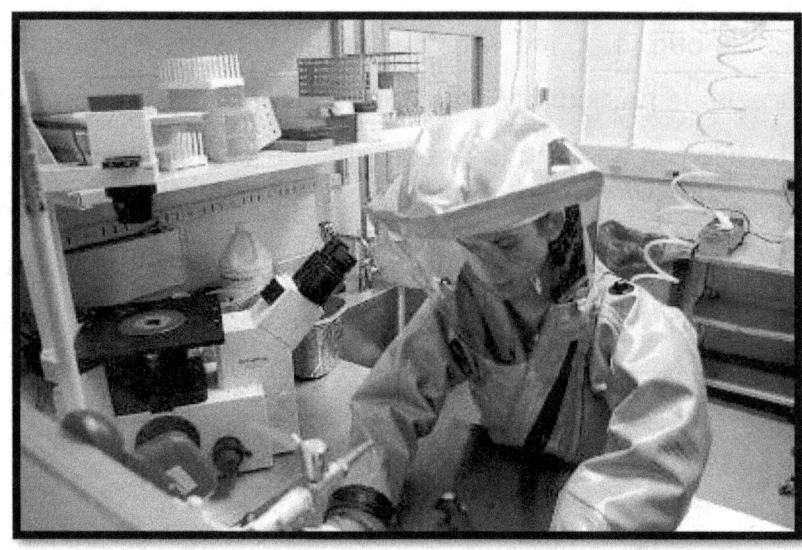

Unless you are a healthcare professional or a friend/family member of an individual who is showing symptoms of Ebola, your risk for exposure is very low. Remember, Ebola is not transmitted by air, water, or food. You cannot catch the disease by simply being in the same room as someone who has either been exposed to the disease or who is showing symptoms themselves. In order to contract the disease, you must ingest or otherwise take into your body the blood or bodily fluids of a person who has Ebola and who is already showing symptoms of the disease. Direct contact with contaminated materials including medical equipment, clothing, needles, and bedding may also put you at risk.

Note: In Africa, there is an additional risk for exposure to Ebola in the handling of bushmeat – that is, wild animals that are hunted for food. Ebola may also be transmitted by direct contact with infected bats.

Treatment for Ebola

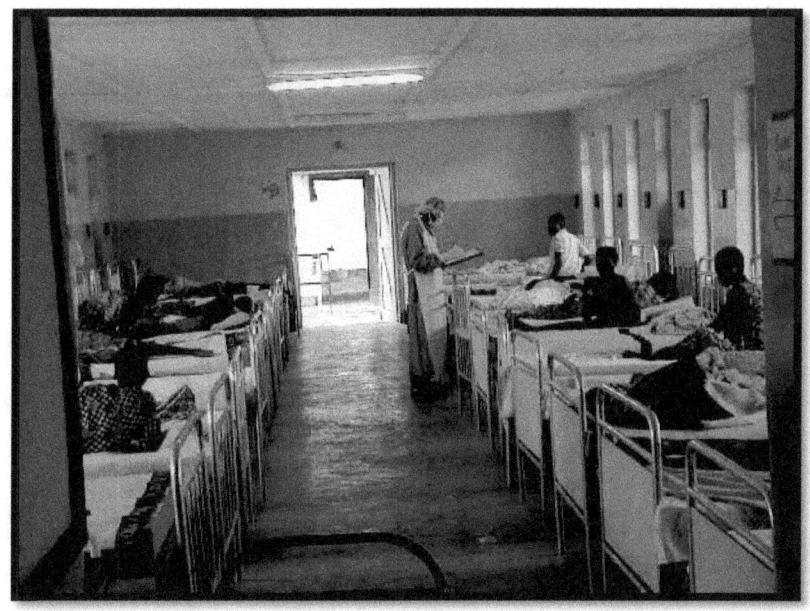

Unfortunately, there is not yet an FDA-approved treatment or vaccine for Ebola. The best medical professionals can do is to treat the symptoms of the disease as they appear. The following treatments are often used for Ebola patients:

- Intravenous (IV) fluids to prevent dehydration and to rebalance electrolytes
- Treatments to maintain blood pressure and oxygen consumption
- Medical treatments for secondary infections, if they occur

The efficacy of these and other treatments for Ebola varies greatly from one patient to another depending on the individual's immune response. Individuals who have a poor immune system are likely to be hit harder by the disease and are less likely to make a full recovery. There are some experimental treatments and vaccines for

Ebola currently being developed, but they have not yet been fully tested for human use. What scientists DO know is that a person who recovers from Ebola develops antibodies against the virus which may be effective for up to 10 years, or more. What scientists do NOT know is whether people who have recovered from Ebola remain immune to the disease for life or if they can later be infected with a different strain. Some individuals who have recovered from the disease carry life-long complications such as joint problems or vision problems.

Prevention of Ebola

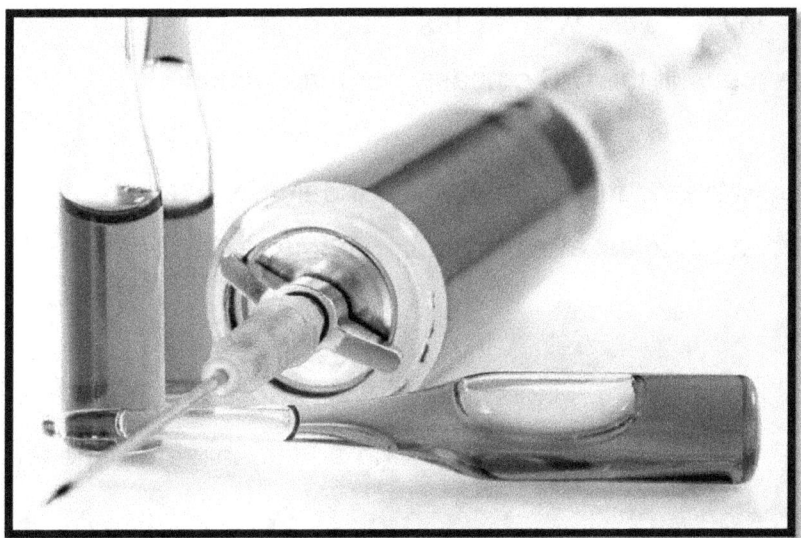

Even though there is no FDA-approved vaccine against Ebola, there are certain things you can do to limit your risk and to prevent the spread of the disease. Some of these prevention methods include:

- Practicing basic hygiene (including washing hands often and avoiding contact with blood and bodily fluids)

- Avoiding contact with items or medical equipment that may have come into contact with an infected person or their blood/bodily fluids

- Do not participate in any funeral or burial practices that involve handling the body of a person who died from Ebola

- Avoid all contact with non-human primates and bats as well as their blood and bodily fluids (including raw meat, if the animals are used as food)

- Do not use any hospitals where Ebola patients are being treated – if you travel to West Africa, consult the U.S embassy for information

- If you travel to West Africa, monitor your health for 21 days after your return and seek immediate medical attention of you begin to develop symptoms

If you are a healthcare worker who may be exposed to patients infected with Ebola, you are encouraged to take the following additional safety measures:

- Always wear the appropriate personal protective gear
- Follow proper sterilization and infection-control measures at all times
- Keep Ebola patients completely isolated from other patients
- Never make direct contact with the blood or bodily fluids of an Ebola patient (including one who has died)
- Contact health care officials if you have had direct contact with the blood, bodily fluids, or contaminated items of an Ebola patient

Past and Present Outbreaks

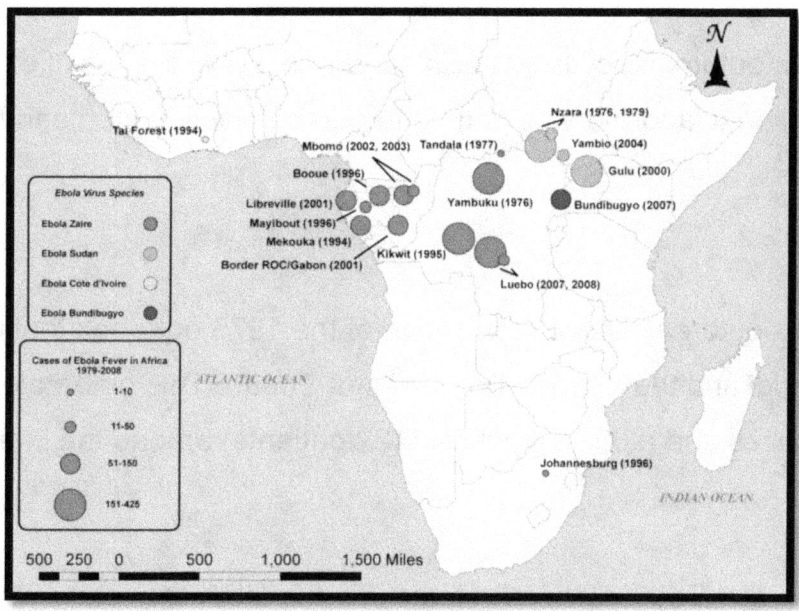

Now that you understand the basics about what Ebola is and how it is spread, you may be curious to know about the past and present outbreaks of the disease. Below you will find a list of some of the most notable Ebola outbreaks in chronological order beginning with the first outbreak that occurred in 1976:

- **1976** – The first outbreak of Ebola occurred in Zaire (the Democratic Republic of Congo), specifically in Yambuku and the surrounding area. The disease is thought to have been spread by close contact with infected patients and by use of contaminated medical equipment. This outbreak resulted in 318 reported cases and an 88% death rate (280 patients) among the infected.

- **1976** – A second outbreak occurred in Sudan in 1976, beginning in Nzara, Maridi and the surrounding areas. This outbreak was caused by close contact with infected patients in a hospital setting and it resulted in 284 reported cases and a 53% death rate (151 patients) among the infected.

- **1976** – This outbreak occurred in England and it was the result of an accidental needle stick in a laboratory setting. One person was infected and recovered from the disease.

- **1979** – This outbreak was a recurrence of the 1976 outbreak that occurred in Nzara, Maridi and the surrounding areas of Sudan. This outbreak resulted in 34 reported cases and a 65% death rate (22 patients) among the infected.

- **1989** – The first Ebola outbreak to occur in the USA happened when the Ebola-Reston virus was introduced by monkeys imported from the Philippines to quarantine facilities in Pennsylvania and Virginia. This outbreak did not infect any humans.

- **1990** - The second USA outbreak occurred in quarantine facilities in Texas and Virginia, spread by monkeys imported from the Philippines. Four human cases were reported – those individuals developed antibodies to the disease but did not develop symptoms.

- **1994** – This outbreak occurred in Mekouka, Gabon, and it affected several gold mining camps in the area. At the time, the disease was diagnosed as yellow fever but was later identified as Ebola hemorrhagic fever in 1995. This outbreak resulted in 52 reported cases and a 60% death rate (31 patients) among the infected.

- **1995** – A second outbreak of Ebola occurred in the Democratic Republic of Congo in the Kikwit area. The outbreak was traced to an index case-patient and was spread through close personal contact by families and in the hospital. This outbreak resulted in 315 reported cases and an 81% death rate (250 patients) among the infected.

- **1996** – Two outbreaks occurred in Gabon during 1996, one in the Boolé area and another in Mayibout area. This outbreak resulted from the consumption of a dead chimpanzee found in the rainforest and was spread by close contact with infected individuals. These outbreaks resulted in 97 reported cases and a 68% death rate (66 patients) among the infected.

- **2000** – This outbreak occurred in the Masindi, Gulu, and Mbarara districts of Uganda, spread by contact with case-patients. This outbreak resulted in 425 reported cases and a 53% death rate (224 patients) among the infected.

- **2001** - Two outbreaks occurred in Gabon during 2001, both on or around the border with the Democratic Republic of Congo. These outbreaks resulted in 122 reported cases and a 79% death rate (96 patients) among the infected.

- **2002** – This outbreak occurred in the Mbomo and Kéllé areas in the Democratic Republic of Congo. This outbreak resulted in 143 reported cases and a 89% death rate (128 patients) among the infected.

- **2007** – This outbreak occurred in the Bundibugyo District of Sudan and it was the first reported occurrence of a new strain of the Ebola virus (the Bundibugyo strain). This outbreak resulted in 149 reported cases and a 25% death rate (37 patients) among the infected.

- **2012** – Two outbreaks occurred during 2012, one in the Kibaale District of Uganda and another in the Orientale Province of the Democratic Republic of Congo. These outbreaks resulted in 47 reported cases and a 36% death rate (17 patients) among the infected.

- **2014** – The largest outbreak of Ebola to date occurred in multiple countries throughout West Africa and the number of patients is currently under investigation. As of November 2014, the patient count was 5481 with a death rate of 54% (2946 patients) among those infected with the disease.

Ebola Q&A

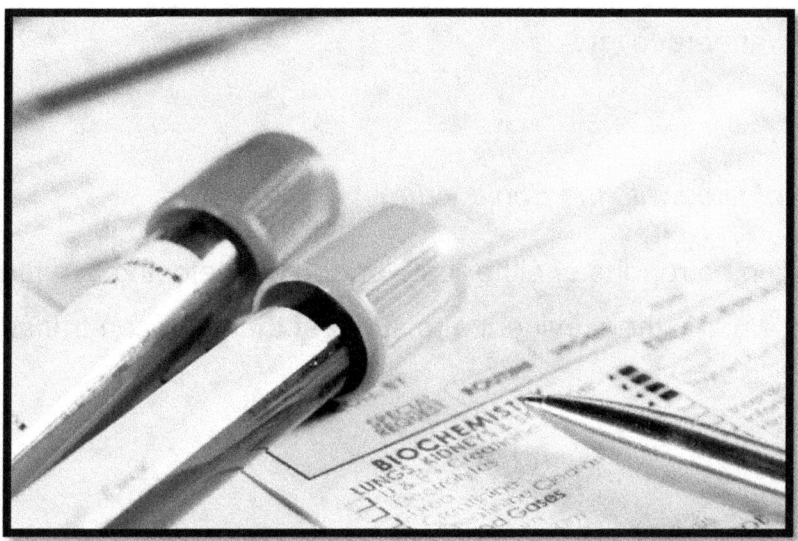

Even after reading this book, you may find that you still have questions about Ebola Virus Disease. In the following pages you will find some commonly asked questions related to the disease as well as their answers:

Q: *Can the Ebola virus be spread through sneezing or coughing?*

A: No evidence has been found to indicate that the disease can be spread through coughing or sneezing. Direct contact with bodily fluids may result in infection, though the disease cannot be spread through the air.

Q: *How long can the Ebola virus live outside the human body?*

A: The virus can only survive on dry surfaces for a few hours and it is easily killed with hospital-grade disinfectant. If the virus is in bodily fluids such as blood, however, it can live for a few days.

Q: *Can a person who survives and recovers from Ebola still spread the disease?*

A: No, a person who has recovered from Ebola is no longer contagious. There is one exception, however. The Ebola virus can still be transmitted through a person's semen for up to 3 months after recovery.

Q: *Can dogs be infected with the Ebola virus?*

A: There have been no reports of either cats or dogs developing symptoms after being exposed to Ebola – nor is there evidence to suggest that they can transmit the disease to humans.

Q: *Can a pet owned by an Ebola patient spread the disease?*

A: It is not yet known whether the paws, fur, or body of a pet can pick up the disease or if it can be spread to other animals or to humans. The CDC recommends that pets owned by an Ebola patient be evaluated by a veterinarian to assess the pet's risk of exposure to bodily fluids or blood.

Q: *Do monkeys spread the Ebola virus?*

A: Yes, it is possible for non-human primates to contract and spread the disease. Primates may exhibit symptoms including fever, reduced appetite, and sudden death. Unless the monkey has been exposed to a person with Ebola, however, they are not at risk for contracting or spreading the disease.

Q: *Can bats spread the virus in the United States?*

A: In Africa, bats are considered the natural reservoir for the Ebola virus but bats in North America are not known to carry the virus.

Conclusion

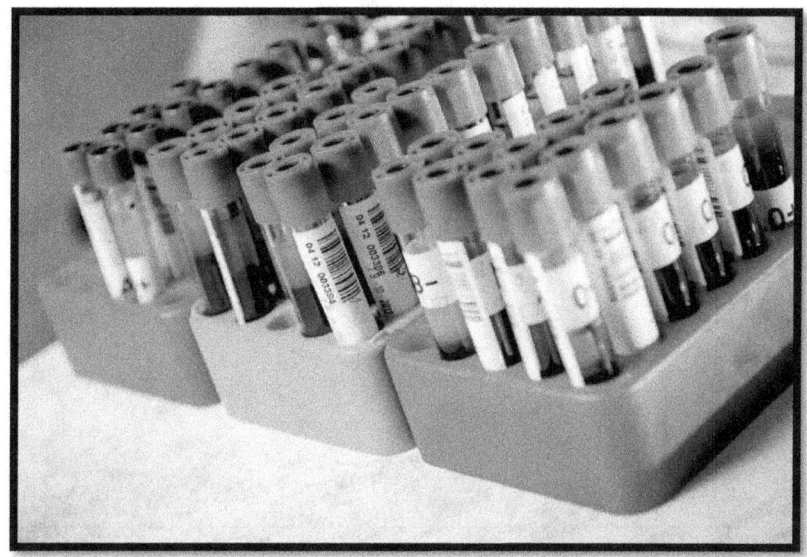

Unfortunately, many people do not realize that Ebola is actually very rare and that your chances of contracting the disease are slim unless you come into direct contact with the blood or bodily fluids of someone showing symptoms of the disease. After reading this book, you should now understand the basics about Ebola including what it is, how it is diagnosed, and what the treatment options are. With this knowledge in hand, hopefully you can help to stop the spread of misinformation and keep your family safe from the disease.

I Need Your Help!

Please take a minute out of your busy schedule to leave a review.

Your review will let readers know what to expect and what you liked about this book. I am looking forward to reading your review.

Thank you so much for your feedback!

How to Submit a Review

To submit a review:

1. Make sure you are signed in.
2. Hover over **Your Account** in the upper right hand corner.
3. Click on **Your Orders**.
4. Click on **Digital Orders**.
5. Click **Write a customer review** in the Customer Reviews section.
6. Rate the item and write your review.
7. Click **Submit**.

How to submit a review from your Kindle device

Please follow the link below for instructions.

http://www.dummies.com/how-to/content/posting-an-amazon-book-review-from-your-kindle.html

Photo Credits

Life Cycle of Ebola by CDC via Wikimedia Commons,
<http://en.wikipedia.org/wiki/File:EbolaCycle.png>

Biosafety Hazard Suit by US Army Medical Research Institute of Infectious Diseases via Wikimedia Commons,
<http://en.wikipedia.org/wiki/File:Biosafety_level_4_hazmat_suit.jpg>

Ebola Outbreak in Uganda by Daniel Bausch via Wikimedia Commons,
<http://en.wikipedia.org/wiki/File:Ebola_outbreak_in_Gulu_Municipal_Hospital.jpg>

Outbreak Map by Zorecchi via Wikimedia Commons,
<http://en.wikipedia.org/wiki/File:EbolaSubmit2.png>

Medical Research by Quintote via Wikimedia Commons,
<http://en.wikipedia.org/wiki/File:Monoclonal_antibodies3.jpg>

Fruit Bat by Staff Sgt. Melissa B. White, via Wikimedia Commons,
<http://commons.wikimedia.org/wiki/File:Mariana_fruit_bat_1.jpg>

Symptoms of Ebola by Mikael Haggstrom via Wikimedia Commons,
<http://en.wikipedia.org/wiki/File:Symptoms_of_ebola.png>